# JUST LIKE THE LOTUS

A Remarkably Honest Account of a Young Girl's Battle with Epilepsy

## CHIARA SPARKS

STOKE Publishing

This book is the personal story of my journey with epilepsy. I offer no medical advice, just my experience. I was 12 when I was diagnosed and completed this book just after my 18th birthday. It is from this perspective that I share my experience.

BULK PURCHASES can be arranged. Please email stokepublishing@hotmail.com directly with your request.

## STAY IN TOUCH!

If you would like to stay up-to-date on what I am doing as I embark on my writing adventures, please sign up here:
https://forms.aweber.com/form/56/63105756.htm

*This book is dedicated to everyone who is struggling right now. There is hope for all of us. Just believe.*

*"Just like the lotus, we too,*
*have the ability to rise from the mud,*
*bloom out of darkness and radiate into the world."*
*Unknown*

*And to Grandpa Frank ... thank you for inspiring me and reminding everyone that I was the smartest one in the litter. Including Dad. Thoughts of you will continue to make me smile. RIP.*

# CONTENTS

# ACKNOWLEDGMENTS

**Sherry Van Hesteren**

Thank you for helping me see that I am on a hero's journey. It has been inspiring to learn that even though I was called to this challenge reluctantly, and given no choice but to cross the threshold into the dark world of struggle, I can overcome. I can write a new ending.

**Matt Burgess**

Thank you for believing in me. Drama has been one of the things that kept me going when I just couldn't anymore.

**Karletta DeWitt**

Thank you for all that you have patiently taught me. You are my role model and I look up to you so much. Riding and horses are such an important part of who I am and your support and understanding is appreciated.

**Dad**

Thank you for understanding how important horses are to

me and for all your support & encouragement along the way. I love you. Let's go see Italy!

**Mom**
You are my everything. You are my right-hand woman, my best friend and my back bone. Thank you for all that you have taught me. You are the perfect Mom for me.
I love you.

# FOREWORD

## By Jennifer Sparks

I am Chiara's mother. On December 31st, 2011, Chiara had her first grand mal seizure, and our lives changed significantly. She was 12 years old at the time. Since then, we've been trying to navigate this new world together. At times, our relationship is dysfunctional and highly codependent, because Chiara sees me as her lifeline, her protector and her tether to what she wants, but can't quite grasp alone. And, of course, I worry about what will happen if I am not there when she needs me. Realistically, I cannot be there every moment of her life, but I am controlled by the need to make sure I am there when *the* moment comes. There have already been moments where she needed me there to protect her, and I missed them. Missing these moments meant no one was there to catch her when she fell. There was no one there to pull the hot curling iron off her face when she seized. There was no one there to protect her face from the concrete she smashed into over and over again by our back step.

Knowing that I need to be there changes the choices we make. It alters both of our personal boundaries. I stay with Chiara more than either of us wants or is healthy. Since we have no way of predicting when one of these moments may arrive, we both feel as though we are held captive by the anxiety and preoccupation of the next seizure. This anticipation has changed the way we move through our days. Each moment of our life looks the same until it doesn't, and this uncertainty creates a sense of fear so thick that some days I cannot breathe.

This disease can easily lead one down a road to absolute overwhelm. It can cripple you. It can tie your mind up in horrible thinking. It can twist your guts. It can mess with your sense of hope, fairness and purpose. It can take away your ability to sleep. It can suck the joy from every single thing. But only if you let it.

Until very recently, Chiara has been dealing with severe anxiety and depression, never knowing when or if another seizure was going to strike her in the middle of what she's trying to make of her life. This has been a difficult journey for her, but she is fighting back. I am in awe of her courage and tenacity. Even on her weakest of days, there is a something I sense within her that tells me this is not what will take her down. It has certainly pushed her to her limits more times than I can say, but she takes the time she needs and then she gets back up, albeit sometimes reluctantly, to keep forging ahead. She still has bad days but she is also having some good ones now.

I know some days she is so incredibly tired. Tired beyond explanation. Tired of everything in a way that none of us will likely ever understand, and on those days, I just do my best to give her every other thing she needs. Some days that thing is love. Some days it is space. Some days it is humour. Some days it is chicken noodle soup. Some days it is an extra day of sleep with no judgement from me, and some days it is a little nudge that she has been down long enough and it is time to do something … anything, other than give up.

Together we have learned that even in hard moments and bad days, there are blessings. Chiara and I have said time and time again that this struggle has brought us a relationship few mother-daughter duos know at this point in a teenager's life. Would we be this close if she was just proceeding along a normal life plan? We both think not, because her medical needs mean she is watched, meds monitored, sleep charted and stresses shared. We fluctuate between being goofy roommates, best friends, annoyed siblings and mother & daughter. As she approaches her 18th birthday, it becomes more and more apparent that I must step back and help her make her way into the world. What that exactly looks like, I have no idea. I just know it is hard, necessary and scary.

Chiara has openly wondered if these lessons could be a chance for her to live a life more true to herself at a much younger age than most. Sickness teaches you great things about living, and many people change their lives when they face a crisis much later in life. Does Chiara get a head start on living authentically? Does this mean she gets to avoid a cancer scare at thirty or a different kind of crisis later in life because she has already learned this lesson? I sure hope so.

Coincidentally, on the fifth anniversary of Chiara's first grand mal seizure, there was an article in our local paper, The StarPhoenix (Dec 31, 2016) written about the local arts scene. Cam Fuller shared that the production that made the biggest impression on him in 2016 was the final performance of The Romeo Project by Persephone's Young Company. Chiara had auditioned for this company because she loves drama and felt that perhaps being on stage would help her overcome anxiety's grip on her. Cam wrote, "I keep coming back to the final performance. The teen cast knocked it out of the park, and Daniel MacDonald's direction gave new insight into the play. But what really topped it was the emotion. The show had to be stopped near the end when one poor girl in the cast had a seizure. After composing themselves, the company came through with a thrilling conclusion to support her and each other. This is what love looks like. There wasn't a dry eye in the house, including mine."

Yes. The girl was Chiara. And today as I write this, I can't help but reflect on the fact that she has never actually *seen* the love and support she receives when epilepsy steals her from us. She was cracked open to something else when she read these words and even though I found her crying, I know she understood a new angle… "This is what love looks like." She is surrounded by it.

While both of us pray that her seizures will become controlled and she will be able to enter life without the worry she carries now, we navigate this not-so-new normal together. We have experienced few highs and many lows. We have relished in some small wins and braced ourselves through some heavy losses. We have hope, and then we don't. We have a new drug, but then it fails. Control for Chiara and her specific condition, Juvenile Absence Epilepsy, has remained elusive. She has tried numerous medications: Keppra, Lamotrigine, Ethosuximide, Vimpat, Brivlera, and CBD oil.

There have been periods where Chiara has had very few seizures, but she has never been seizure free. We have also tried a modified Adkins diet (MAD), energy healing, naturopathic medicine, homeopathic medicine, energy work and other alternative healing approaches. Some have produced improvements, and others have not.

Her diagnosis has shifted my perception of wellness significantly. It has become a passion of mine, in part because I feel the more I know, the more I can help her. But what I am quickly learning is this is her battle, and she has been called to the front line alone. I can support her, but I can't fight her battle. I can't trade places. I can't buy her health. And some days it kills me to have to witness any of it.

As a mother, it is a horrible thing to watch your child suffer and to see years of youth vaporized in a drug-induced fog, or to know some of her best memories or most exciting opportunities are messed up, erased or contaminated by seizures. Or to stare her in the eyes and see nothing but wide-open eyes and a vacant look when I ask her if she knows who I am. Sometimes I can see her panic, and with no ability to communicate at that moment, I can see her locked inside. I know that even my reassuring words do not get to her in these moments and I hate that I know she is afraid.

Someone asked me if I felt like I had lost my daughter to

this disorder and the medication side effects. My answer is a heartbroken yes. One night a beautiful, vivacious, life-loving 12-year-old went to sleep, and had I known that would be the last time I would see that version of her, I would have held her tightly and never let her go.

Yes, I have been waiting for her to come back to me. I am waiting for her to find her laughter and joy again. I am waiting for her energy to lift her from her bed and back into her life full force. I am waiting... but in my heart, I now know I will never again see my 12-year-old daughter, because these past five years have stolen that child from me. These past five years have stolen from her the chance to develop and explore possibilities in a carefree manner. Five years have vaporized in a blur.

The drugs, the sedation, the seizures, the mood swings, the rage, the sorrow and the frustration buried her normal development. I wish so badly I could have witnessed as my daughter grew from a teenager into a young woman. Instead, this all happened behind a veil of overwhelm and struggle. The 12-year-old child is gone, but I am still waiting for the joyful, vivacious and fun-loving young lady to make her way home. I see glimpses. I know she is there. I have hope I will meet her one day.

As I write this, Chiara has been stable for the first time in a long time. We had a scary ordeal in October, and it forced our hand to try another medication change with a new doctor in charge of her care. Dare we hope that THIS is her last dance with this disease? She has finally been able to get off Keppra without dropping within twelve hours from a seizure. I can already see a significant change in her mental health. The darkness is lifting. She is engaged more in life and with people. Friends and family see a change too. I hear her laughing, and I notice it because I realize now how absent it has been. But still, it is up and down.

We know that in sharing our story, our struggles, our vulnerability, our breakdowns and our breakthroughs, we might be helping somebody else out there make it to the next day. Chiara's words, explanations and perspectives may help another parent understand what their child is facing when they are unable to communicate that them-selves. Perhaps, as a parent, I will be able to offer some guidance to others who are struggling to deal with what we are dealing with, someone who is a few steps behind me, looking for a little guidance to find their way out of the overwhelm. I know that hope can be cruel, but I also know that it can change the way you function.

Chiara is an incredibly strong and resilient young woman. She is also very tender and caring. She deals with things on a daily basis that most people will never experience in their lifetime. If there was anything I could do to take away her heartbreak and give her back the time and experi-ences that epilepsy has stolen from her life, I would.

But as we have learned, we are often not in control of our lives as much as we think we are. As we cannot control what's happening here, we have to lean towards controlling how we react to situations and events. Some days, this is easier for me than others. Some days, Chiara takes the lead, and some days, we both come crashing down together. In all of this, I've learned that when I'm open and honest about what we're struggling with, people reach out to support us. Chiara has some amazing friends. Epilepsy has helped her sort those true gems from the rest of the noise.

Chiara is wise beyond her years. She can sense struggle in people and is driven to provide comfort. She is empathetic in a way that I have not seen many people be. Chiara is an amazingly intuitive girl. She is learning in her struggle, and it is our greatest hope that this book project is going to allow her to rewrite her story and to change the ending once and for all.

# ORDINARY ME

*"Never own a disease. Reduce the amount of time that you will talk about being ill. Refuse to allow illness a place in your consciousness." - Synchronicities of The Universe*

My mother would describe me as a risk taker. I was always sneaking out the back door of the house and venturing out on escapades in the neighbourhood looking for animals. I would slip out when she was busy and make my way down the street to the house where I knew a dog lived. I would knock on the door and ask if the dog could come out and play. I didn't really care to play with other children if animals were around. I loved nature and animals in general, but above all I loved horses.

I would ride my bike for hours in the summer, zipping off on imaginary adventures, with nothing but a few sweaty coins squeezed in my fist for a drink half way through the day. I would hop off my bike while it was still moving. I would come home exhausted and fall asleep satisfied that I had lived the day the best I could. Mom said I was fiercely independent and feared very little. She said I had a good head on my shoulders and she didn't have to worry too much about me.

I enjoyed school for a few years, but I was slow to learn to read. Once I did catch on though, I was a pretty good student. Mom never had to ask me to get stuff done; I just did it. I enjoyed it. I had some great friends.

I've spent the first week of every July since I was four years old camping just outside of Saskatoon with my childhood friends, and these are some of my most treasured memories.

In summer, our family would also go north to our cabin and I would swim care-freely in the deep, cold northern lakes. I learned to skinny-dip up there. I would wake up at 5 a.m. to go fish off the dock, because I was determined to catch a lake monster... Lac La Beast, we called it. I learned to catch frogs and leaches. I enjoyed the late night campfires and marshmallow s'mores. Life was simple.

I barely remember what it feels like to be that girl. I do know life didn't feel heavy at the time, as it does now. That girl feels so far away. She is almost a stranger now.

Looking back, I guess I have described a typical childhood; I lived in an ordinary world. My mom and brother and I had some awesome family vacations, swimming in the ocean in Hawaii and Mexico, and we explored California together with a faulty GPS and a true sense of adventure. ***Life was routine but predictable, and I have learned that there is freedom in predictability, too.*** If you know what to expect, you can do many things.

I try to keep epilepsy separate from my identity. I am not

epilepsy and it is not me. But this disease can be intrusive in all areas of your life. The separation between disease and person becomes increasingly difficult if the battle has been a long and unsuccessful one. Disease can be all-consuming. It can swallow you whole. I can't pretend it isn't pulling me down.

Perhaps the most important thing right now is understanding that each day is a fresh start. Some days, that feels like all the hope I have. Other days, I have no hope at all, but I know that tomorrow will still arrive, and if it doesn't arrive, well, then I guess nothing matters anyway.

### Epilepsy

so many layers of dysfunction
it can't really be explained
or understood
Yet
epilepsy is just a word
a word that knows how to throw a party of
migraines, sore muscles, tears
eventually it changes

It moves from
'I have epilepsy' to
'I am epilepsy'

It becomes mental and emotional
over time

Pain
Is no longer just physical
waking from a seizure
regaining awareness, speech, sanity

I'm not worried about me
I don't care that
I am hurting physically
that every single muscle in my body feels torn
that the acid from my vomit
has set my throat on fire
that I bite my tongue and
that my lungs are full of my most recent meal
I don't care.
It's unfair and it hurts but
I don't care.

What hurts is waking up and knowing
you are still epilepsy.
Disappointment.
What hurts is
seeing your mother's tear-stained cheeks
hearing that your dad came to the hospital to see you and
was rubbing your temples to help your pain
but you have no recollection of
his love and concern.

A father that you desperately need.
A father that you would never send away unless you were
incoherent and coming out of a seizure

Epilepsy controls life
it becomes who you are
It begins to define you

Epilepsy has stolen my teenage years.
It has taken away time I should have had
to grow and figure out who I am.
It took away opportunity and then it took its place
Epilepsy has scarred my body and soul
but I will not break.
I am not epilepsy.
I am Chiara and
Chiara I will remain.

# How did this all begin?

It began, oddly enough, with waffles. I was making waffles with my father, brothers and step-mom one morning. Apparently, I was stirring the batter and my dad called me to grab the milk. I wasn't answering, and he thought I was just being a smart ass because I wasn't replying. Eventually, they realized something was wrong with me. I was having a seizure standing up. I don't remember much about it. But this was the foggy beginning of a new life for me, even if I didn't realize it at the time. Actually, it was the beginning of less life for me.

They put me on the couch and I woke up to my dad trying to make me eat waffles. He was trying to stick food in my mouth, trying to get me to eat, because he didn't know that it was a seizure. He thought maybe it was a blood sugar thing. That was my very first identified seizure and, as we would come to learn, I was having 30 or more a day. We were unaware of this, because they were fleeting and hard to catch when life was going on around you.

What you will learn as I share my story is that because epilepsy steals your memories and your brain function, if you have ever been with me when I had a seizure you already know more than I do. I think it is hard for people to understand what a seizure does to the brain and your ability to function. You look the same, so it is hard to really understand that everything has changed.

Scrambled brain. Scrambled memories. Scraps. Days later things may slide back together but it is never complete. There are always pieces of the puzzle missing. It's like a jigsaw puzzle you are so excited to finish, and when you get to the last piece in the box, you see there is still a gaping hole left in the puzzle and you have no more pieces in sight.

Yeah, good luck finding the last pieces. Incomplete. Everything is left incomplete.

# LIFE INTERUPTED

## You can't pretend it never happened.

*I* guess my journey really began when I had my first full grand mal seizure on December 31, 2011, because prior to that we knew something weird was happening, but we didn't know what that was.

When I had the grand mal it set a few things into motion. You can't miss these ones because everything literally stops. Even breathing. Unlike some of the other seizures, this one you can't ignore. You can't pretend it never happened. You can't go on with life. They just rip the world out from underneath your feet. No warning.

My mother tells me that the first seizure she witnessed is burned into the backs of her eyelids so much that she can't blink the memory away. I know she thought I was actually dead when she saw me. She can describe in fine detail everything that took place. The fear she felt then she still carries with her. It is something she struggles with a lot of the time.

I don't really remember anything other than the paramedic. I remember her blonde hair and her blue eyes and just how pretty she was and then it hit me, two minutes later, as to why there were paramedics in my house. I think I knew in my heart what had happened before I knew it in my head.

J ennifer:

This story really begins on December 31, 2011. Chiara was twelve years old at the time. This was the day that she had her first grand mal seizure. She had a friend sleep over and they were up the next day having breakfast in front of the TV when I went to go and have a shower. Shortly after I stepped under the water, her friend was pounding on the bathroom door telling me that something was wrong with Chiara. When I came in to the living room, I found my daughter on the floor, grey, frothing at the mouth, with her hands and wrist contorted and twisted into her chest. She was not breathing and in that moment, I truly thought that I had lost her. Little did I know that this was the beginning of a very long journey for us and everyone who loves her.

Looking back now, I believe that her petit mal seizures probably started sometime in the fall of 2011, then progressed into grand mal seizures in December. She was twelve years old when this all started. She is now almost eighteen and until five months ago, we had yet to find an acceptable way to control her seizures. She was having both petit mal and grand mal seizures and her last grand mals ended up putting her in the hospital for five days.

She is on Lamotrigine, Brivlera, Ethosuximide, and we have been exploring the use of CBD Oil to control her seizures. We finally just dropped the last 250 mg of Keppra and it has made a long overdue positive impact on her mental health. She was on 3000mg a day, but I started weaning her off awhile back. This drug has always caused issues and truly changed my daughter in so many ways. It just became intolerable.

She also has anxiety and depression as a result of the diagnosis and the changes to her lifestyle, energy levels and ability to cope with life. Chiara has had seizures on the backs of horses, on theatre stages, in class, in the hallways at school and home, on high bar stools, at the kitchen table, in mid-sentence, reaching to close a window, in the car, while doing homework, while driving, while walking and while bathing. Life interrupted over and over again. How do you live fully when uncertainty is in your face?

One of the biggest battles has been the side effects from the medications. Just a note upfront about medications. They work differently for everyone, so keep that in mind when we share her side effects. Don't avoid a drug because of what you may learn here, just be aware. Every case is different.

Keppra has induced a fair amount of rage. Lamotrigine has been fairly easy to adapt to, but she's on a very high dose that causes joint pain. Vimpat gave her double vision, so we stopped that when she had trouble negotiating the hallways. Keppra was the first drug she was put on and we tried for years to wean her off of the Keppra entirely, but each time she had a grand mal seizure within twelve hours.

After her last hospital stay her new doctor helped get her off Keppra once and for all! We celebrated that week. That was one of our wins.

We have taken her to the Mayo Clinic, tried energy healing, Reiki, chiropractic, massage, diet, but we are still not done trying. My goal is to get my daughter's seizures controlled and reinstate a quality of life into her daily living. What will her adult life look like? What kind of work can she do? How will she pay for these medications? How can we make sure she is safe and healthy AND independent.

I wanted to address something that I've heard time and time again. When people learn Chiara has petit mal seizures, they assume it is not a real problem. The petit mal, or absence seizures, are sometimes hard to see. They are usually short in duration, but they can have a tremendous impact on her ability to function. I've had people say to me, "Oh, the little seizures. That's not a big deal," but it is a big deal. Can you just imagine knowing your operating system is going to fail you, but you don't know when? What if you were flying a plane and the engine had a habit of quitting without warning? What if you're riding a bicycle and you check out for 10 seconds? Will you drive that bicycle into traffic? Will you drive it into a tree? Will you veer of into something more dangerous? A life can change dramatically in ten seconds. Ten seconds can be a big deal.

Chiara has EEG tests that revealed she was having over 30 petit mals in a 24-hour period. This is a problem. It's a big problem, and when people tell her it's not a problem, it's extremely frustrating for her.

I'd like you to imagine for a moment that you're a computer, and I'm going to unplug you a hundred times today. How do you think your memory will be impacted? How do you think your productivity will be impacted? How do you think your engagement will be impacted? Your mood? Your desire to try new thing? Petit mals are a big deal, even if it's just 10 seconds or 20 seconds at a time. And, often, the petit mals grow into the grand mals.

Truly gaining a seizure-free life would mean Chiara would be able to live her life with no seizure activity whatsoever, and, in conjunction with that, we would like her to be able to cope more effectively with the side effects from the medications that she's taking.

We have found that Chiara's very sensitive to medication, and as such, she has some issues tolerating the side effects, which are tremendously hard on her. One is sedation. With the whole goal of stopping the excitable brain, Chiara has been sedated to a point where, at times, she has slept up to 20 hours a day. A child, a growing child, an adolescent, a teenager that is sleeping 20 hours a day is not going to be a happy person. Not to mention when you sleep that much, there is an impact on your muscles and your ability to move through life with some degree of stamina. It redefines what a "normal day" looks like. In addition, she's often dizzy. She has sight issues. She has memory issues, and she has nausea. And then she has people saying it is not a big deal.

We don't have an option to ignore this condition. Instead we have learned to try to manage what we can control and focus on that instead.

# YEAH, HOW ABOUT WE DON'T GO THERE

*D*id you have any idea, at the time of your first seizure, what the next five years of your life would be like?

No. I figured we would get a medication and it would be problem solved. I had no idea what other things might come into play. I would never have even considered how the medication would make me feel. I think I just wanted to believe this was going to be no big deal at all. Just give me the meds and I will be fine. Even at 12, I knew doctors gave pills that fixed things so they could just do that for me.

**How has the last five years actually evolved for you?**

It's been full of anxiety, depression, sadness, anger and even rage. Grief too. The last five years of my life haven't played out the way that five-year-old me would have assumed that my teenage years would. I had no idea that a life could be turned upside down like this without warning. I had never really thought about not living a great life.

**You're going to take your reader on a journey with you over the last five years. When they come to the end of this book, are they going to learn a lesson? Is there going to be a bigger picture of hope here for them to hang onto?**

I don't know if there's going to be a big lesson, because I'm still learning my lessons as I go. I am also not sure you can always recognize lessons AS you are learning them. I think we need to reflect on things and step back a bit to pick out the pieces that are meaningful for that to happen.

I don't think I have had that single big lesson in all of this. I think that I've learned some little lessons, like what a good friend is, or how to be more compassionate, but this journey that epilepsy has taken me on I don't think is over. I don't think it's anywhere near over. I think that writing this book might help me grow in some ways, because I have to think harder about all of this stuff I would rather avoid thinking about at all.

While I don't think there's going to be one big lesson learned in the end, I hope at some point I can string all the little lessons together into something that makes sense. I feel like right now, I am still too close to the details to be able to step back and look at the state my life has become, and not feel totally emotionally overwhelmed. It is hard to learn when you are drowning in emotions you can't process. Stay with me, maybe we will all be surprised in the end. Maybe I know more than I think I do already.

Maybe I assume that people know more than they do. Maybe I can help someone else see things differently. I guess you get to be the judge of what you learn from me.

## I DON'T KNOW MY WAY

"The symbol of the lotus flower gives a precious teaching that can inspire us to deal with life in the best possible way. Its roots take nourishment from muddy waters and yet bloom in full delicacy and beauty on the surface. Similarly, to have a positive mindset is a beautiful quality, nonetheless to be transformational it needs to be rooted firmly in reality to then blossom with the value which can be created from the muddy problem." - Dorotea Brandin

My mom went to an Epilepsy support meeting and told me she cried for two hours straight in a room full of people who understood exactly what she was feeling without having to explain the little details that other people need explained. It was such a relief for her to be able to let go and she wished she had gone years ago, because it felt so good to just be with people that understood all elements of our struggle without having to explain it. She really wants me to go to one of the next meetings, but I am not at all interested.

She told me about some awesome people she met but I am not sure I even care. I'm too tired to care.

There was a young lady there named Carmen who was married to a really great guy, and they were expecting their

first baby. The young lady's mom, Caroline, was there too
and my mom felt connected to them both. She told me
Carmen said she would meet with me for coffee anytime
because she has a very similar story to mine, but she is ten
years ahead of me in her process. I didn't know when my
mom told me about these people, that someday I would be
sitting in a restaurant wanting to die, looking across the
table at them for hope. And they would give it to me.

I met Carmen and her mother, Caroline, at the mall for
coffee. My mom had arranged it because she knew I was
on the verge of slipping into the darkness, and nothing she
was saying to me was getting into my head. I sat there,
with the cuts on my arms hidden beneath my sleeves,
listening to Carmen's words, knowing she understood all
that I couldn't say.

I cried and they listened. Carmen told me about her
struggle and about her happy life with her first baby due
any day now. There is hope but fuck, I hate this. I hate not
knowing how long I have to struggle before I can take a
deep breath and know I will be okay.

That meeting changed things for me. I now had a place to
go in my head when things were hard. I now had another
story to compare my own things to, and I felt supported. I
knew I was not alone. I knew that others had struggled and
won. Others just like me. I think in one meeting, I realized
that the support from those who had been there and who
actually KNOW what it is like is crucial. We need to know
it is okay to reach out for help, and it is freeing to accept
help from those who offer it. They want to give it.

Those who have fought a battle similar to yours can give

you insight. They know what you are going to feel next, even before you do. They can warn you and prepare you. They can explain it in a way you really understand. They can provide tips for surviving, because they had to fight to learn them firsthand. I knew after that meeting that I still had a long way to go, but … I also knew I was not alone. I knew there was hope.

# LOST AT SEA

**a poem**

My life with epilepsy
like a ship lost at sea.
A grand, old fashioned ship
setting off on its maiden voyage
to a new world
with such hope, excitement, possibilities.
Instead
eventually finding itself shredded to bits
struggling towards foreign shores

A ship lost at sea ...
The first of many colossal waves hits,
nearly tipping the ship over

The second wave strikes the front of the ship,
blinding the Captain who can no longer steer
Water has covered the ship's deck,
waves twisting
drowning hope, choking

Everyone on board loses their balance,
a few fall overboard
The Captain
now back on his feet
guides the ship as best he can
but remains blinded by the
ocean's angry spray
and the darkness of a cloudy, heavy night.
Not even the North Star can guide him now.
Despair

The key is to keep calm isn't it?
Keep calm for whom?
It won't help the crew and
it won't stop the storm.
Relentless

All direction is lost,
the world is draped in darkness.
It cloaks its predators and feeds regret.
If only …

Hardly any ship left
A grand ship on its maiden voyage
to a new world,
sinking before the foreign shores.
Incomplete voyage

Sinking,
struggling,

shoreline approaching.
Hope within grasp.

If only I could fly
away

## NO CHOICE BUT ALL IN

"The flower that blooms in adversity is the most rare and beautiful of all." - Unknown

**W**hat is it like when you have a seizure?

I don't really know. I do not have any warning or auras. It doesn't hurt, but I know it must look pretty scary because I can sense the fear in people, and in some ways I am socially excluded, because people worry it will happen when they are around. I wake up looking at unfamiliar things and people. Sometimes I can hear, but not speak properly. I know time has passed but have no idea how much time. It feels like you are locked inside your own body, unable to communicate. Parts of my brain work, but things do not connect. Coming out of a seizure is like trying to climb out of quicksand, and the more you struggle and fight it, the harder it is.

**J**ennifer:

Since Chiara loses consciousness, I will share with you what I have seen.

Every seizure is different. If the seizure has attacked a particular part of her brain, it can take a really long time for her to realize who she is, where she is and what's happened. Sometimes, she'll lose a tremendous amount of memory on either side of the seizure. Other times, she loses very little. She has lost entire days. She has asked me to stop lying to her when I explain we have done something she can't recall. Every event is a bit different. If she is having petit mals and I am not aware, she may keep asking the same questions over and over. If I say I already told you about this or that and she says that I did not, then I know that something is likely going on that I am not seeing. Anytime I hear my inside voice question her behavior, I know I need to watch her more closely.

When she first starts to come-to after a grand mal seizure, she doesn't know where she is and she's extremely confused. She doesn't recognize anybody who's around her, even if she's known them for years. She mumbles and tries to speak but can't. She looks at me like she doesn't know me. Her eyes are either empty or panic-stricken. She can seem almost child-like. She can be angry or loving. It's a toss-up as to how it all rolls out.

This post-ictal phase can last anywhere from fifteen or twenty minutes, to up to an hour. If she doesn't seem to be able to make sense after that time, we go to ER to make sure she is okay. With her last grand mal in October, she never fully recovered from it and then had another grand mal follow. She needed medical intervention to get things under control again. Then an allergic reaction to the IV medication complicated matters. She ended up staying in the hospital for five days to sort things out.

Sometimes, she will awaken very afraid of where she is and try to stand, but she's not able to keep her balance and she stumbles around almost like she's intoxicated. As a parent, my biggest concern is that she'll have a grand mal seizure somewhere and then people will see her stumbling around confused and out of it and think that she's been doing drugs or she's intoxicated, and she'll be treated differently or ignored, when in fact she is experiencing a medical emergency.

When Chiara has a grand mal seizure, she stops breathing for the duration of the actual convulsions. Many times, she will begin to turn blue. When the convulsions stop, it takes a few moments before she begins breathing again on her own. Her seizures last anywhere from about ninety seconds to three minutes, and these moments can truly be the longest moments of my life. If you ever find someone seizing, roll them into the recovery position to keep them from aspirating and banging their head, then get medical attention. Do not try to put anything in their mouth because it can make things worse and you don't want your fingers in there if the jaw clamps down. Trust me! If they recover and try to wander off, keep a close eye on them until they have fully recovered or medical help has arrived.

Many times I have to tell Chiara again and again what's happened until it kind of sticks in her head. She will ask the same questions over and over again with no recollection that we have just had a conversation about what she is asking. It is like Groundhog Day over and over again.

For me, I find it heartbreaking to continually have to break the news that she's had another seizure, or that something's happened on the stage at one of her plays, or that she was on her horse and had a seizure. Every time she asks, I have to explain again and watch her heart break. Then we repeat the process. For me, that's the hardest part, because I don't watch her heart break once, I have to watch it break over and over and over again. I watch as she puts all the pieces together and can see the disappointment and heartbreak all over her face.

Then silence follows, and she retreats into her head. I can't go with her, so I never really know what she is thinking, but it feels sad and heavy and dark.

she falls
unknowingly
wakes broken
hurt & bruised
surrenders momentarily
to her grief
and then
rises again

I find that many people don't or are unable to understand that she is extremely disconnected from her body, and that while she looks the same, her behavior is erratic and so out of character. Often, she will swear repeatedly and she'll be in looped statements or conversations that just repeat themselves over and over again. Many times, I have initially though she was kidding or pulling a prank only to realize it was the onset of a seizure.

If you come across her after she's had her seizure, you may

find her in a post-ictal phase talking or babbling about something, but not making any sense at all. It's just really important that as a friend, you keep her safe and out of harm's way until she begins to come back into her awareness and also to reach out for help if you think you need it. I tell all of Chiara's friends that when in doubt, they can call 911 and get medical staff on site, and that I will deal with what takes place after that. I think this goes for any person who has a seizure.

As a parent, it's very scary to let your child go out into the world to try to be normal, try to do all the things that teenagers want to be able to do knowing full well that if something like this happens, people may freak out and take off because they are frightened by what's taking place. It can be scary if you don't know what's happening and you don't know what to do. It is scary even when you do know what is happening!

My greatest fear is that somebody will leave her because they will think that she has over dosed on drugs or is mentally unstable. I always think about how a seizure event could play out on public transportation, for example. Or I worry that if she is with her peers and they're doing something that they shouldn't be doing (teen stuff) and she has an issue, people will panic and take off, leaving her without the people around to support and care for her when she needs it the most. As a parent, the scariest thing is sending her out in the world knowing that I'm depending fully on the public at large to help keep her safe and bring her home to me each night.

# Chiara:

So I guess I don't have any options here. I am all in. I am all in and at war with my own brain.

# ICED TEA

## A Poem

It used to be my favourite drink.
I loved the sweet lemon-kissed aftertaste it left in
my mouth.
But I rarely drink iced tea anymore because each time I do,
that aftertaste on my tongue digs up memories
I am trying to bury, to forget.

I remember waking after a seizure
with that sweet taste in my mouth
Mixed with my own blood, it took me a while
to figure out the oddly familiar aftertaste
was subtly disguised by blood.
I was continuously swallowing
to try to process my confusion.

When I finally came to and returned to reality,
I realized that I had spilled my once favourite drink all
over myself.
It was sticky and frozen to me.

I was outside and it was -30C when my brain decided it
would be a good idea to spaz out and dump liquid all over.
Death by iced tea.
I rarely drink my iced tea anymore.
It makes me  think of how precious my life is
and it reminds me of how weak I am.

## BAD DAYS & CONSTANT BATTLES

"The lotus is the most beautiful flower, whose petals open one by one. But it will only grow in the mud. In order to grow and gain wisdom, first you must have the mud – the obstacles in life and its suffering. The mud speaks of the common ground that humans share, no matter what our stations in life...Whether we have it all or we have nothing, we are all faced with the same obstacles: sadness, loss, illness, dying and death. If we are to strive as human beings to gain more wisdom, more kindness, and more compassion, we much have the intention to grow as a lotus and open each petal one by one." - Goldie Hawn

**W**hat is a bad day like for you, Chiara?

A bad day with epilepsy, generally ... It's hard to tell, because I have severe depression and anxiety, so the epilepsy, when it mixes in, creates this tornado of awful emotion. A bad day would often go like this:

I'd wake up feeling beyond exhausted, my eyes would hardly open. I can't move my body physically, it feels like I literally cannot move. My heart hurts, just from the exhaustion alone. The sadness is overwhelming. I can physically feel my sadness. I know that on really bad days, there's been times where I collapse because I'm so sad. I can't actually hold myself up, so I collapse. I just start crying because that's what you do when you're sad. I have little breakdowns. Obviously I'm crying and curled up in a ball. A bad day is ... bad.

And good days, I don't really remember what good days feel like. Honestly, a good day would consist of not having a seizure, or not having this heavy feeling of the drugs pushing me into a hole that I can't push back against. A good day for me would really be simple. I would just like to be me. Whoever I am now. I am not really sure anymore. I think some days I do not even know when I had a good day. I am just kind of shut off.

**Visualize Something Better**

My mom asks me to dream about what my perfect day would be like, if I could have one right now. I know she asks me to imagine better things because she believes we become what we think about. So I try…

I wake up. I don't have depression or anxiety or epilepsy. I can go out and ride my horse. It's sunny, it's nice. There are clouds so it's not too hot and not too cold. Just that perfect day. There's a little breeze, there's no bugs, I'll ride my horse out in the field and we can run around and play and be carefree. No anticipation of anything going wrong. I like it when it's just me and Whisper, my horse, because I like hanging out with her. She calms me. I love the smell of her. I know she will keep me safe. After my ride, I would come home, cuddle on the couch with my dog, Rolo, and ... and then I run out of ideas, because I have such a limited amount of experience with good days and few clear memories now of who I used to be.

The thing is, I don't remember what life is like without depression, so I don't know what happiness really feels like. I feel like I am stumbling in the dark when I am asked to imagine that.

The last time I was really happy and excited about something, I fired up my brain and had a seizure. It doesn't even feel safe for me to try happy on.

My mom presses me a bit. Feel it Chiara, smell it, taste it, hear it, see it … what does it feel like for your entire body?

Bliss. On my horse racing the barrels. Free. Focused. Not the ideal hobby for an epileptic, but taking away riding and horses would be about the same as taking away my ability to breathe.

It feels so great on the days I can actually escape this life, using my imagination to go wherever I want. I know I tell my mom it isn't that I don't want to go to school, it is that I can't. I literally cannot.

**So Let's Talk About School**

School fucking sucks. What do I like about school? I like that I get to see my friends every now and then, and the teachers are very supportive for the most part. The drama teacher and the resource room teacher especially, and the former principal, they're all very nice. The new principal doesn't seem to get it at all. You know when you can just sense when it is not even worth trying to make someone understand something because you know they actually lack the ability to understand? I have learned not to bother. Educators can make ALL the difference and many of mine made a positive impact on my situation.

For the most part, I don't talk to other teachers. But I can tell you that a good teacher can make all the difference. There's some EA's that I really love, too, but everything else I'm not really a fan of. I am not sure that people fully understand what it actually takes for me to physically get to school. Many days I get up and get ready and then I just can't make it out the door. Once I am at school, I try to be engaged because I do really love learning but the drug fog can be very heavy. I can be sitting in my chair over-whelmed with the fear that something will happen or I can be sitting there wrestling with the pull of sleep. If my body feels funny in any way I begin to get paranoid something is about to happen. Sitting and listening is very difficult.

Overcrowded classrooms are also worrying. They get so hot in the warmer weather (we have no AC in my school) and when I get overheated bad things happen. I can't even convince myself entering a room that is hot and full of people is a good idea. I had a seizure in a room like that. It is like there is a barrier at the door I cannot cross.

I love drama, but I wish we didn't need to be marked. I wish we could just do it all for the fun of it. The expecta-tions for what I can achieve are different and memorizing lines is so hard for me. I do it for hours. I get angry at my brain for betraying me. I enjoy drama, but I still struggle in a different way in drama. Drama provides other things too. Because drama is so social and active it is easier to stay engaged. I also get to pretend to be someone other than myself. It can be a welcome break from reality. My drama teacher is awesome too and I know he has my back. He also had seen my seizure on stage and was more than willing to help me. He made me feel safe.

I don't like going to school for a million reasons, but when I think about how far behind I am, it frustrates me. If my brain would cooperate, I would be able to do well in school. I hate that I can't show that. Moving some of my classes online has helped because I can work at my own pace and not feel left behind.

When I go to the front office there's the, "warning kids list," kids that have medical issues or concerns and I hate seeing my face on there, knowing that most people don't have a problem that people need to be on alert for. It bothers me that I'm almost an adult and people constantly have to look out for me. A normal 17-year-old doesn't have to be constantly watched. They don't. It's aggravating and it pisses me off, but I know that people are just trying to help. Sometimes it's just suffocating that people are so concerned, but the alternative is equally uncomfortable. I feel like I'm being smothered and I can't breathe, and I want to learn how to be independent, and people aren't letting me be independent because they're too scared.

The only thing I like about school is seeing my friends, and I don't have that many friends because I attend so infrequently. I have acquaintances and people I get along with, but I don't have friends. Not having friends in my classes is an anxiety trigger for me. What if I have to do a group project? I'm going to be paired up with people I don't know and I can't do that. I just can't. Thankfully, my cousin Jack is in some of my classes this term. He is so helpful and awesome and he makes me laugh. He understands because he knows me in and out of school.

My memory also sucks. Some days, nothing sticks at all. It

is very hard to pay attention when you can't recall a
conversation. I feel stupid and I get scared that I will say
something that makes me look like an idiot. I know it is
the drugs that makes my ability to remember things so
poor. I used to have an amazing memory, so I know it's
not me.

I guess it is important for teachers to know that they can
make a difference. My learning plan is modified to account
for my memory issues, which helps take the pressure off
me to memorize things I can always look up. Presenting
class projects can be an issue, because I worry I will seize
at the front of the class. I also worry about not being able
to find my words or looking stupid. I like knowing my
teacher has my back, but not in an oppressive way. It helps
make me feel safe but still more normal.

My teachers have been flexible and supportive, and it
helps. I would have dropped out of school completely had
they not been so awesome. Taking the online classes has
also been key to getting through school because it allows
me to learn when I am well and rest when I am not. I think
part of the success with school comes with letting go of
what might be a normal plan. That is not an easy thing to
do for anyone.

**Medications**

Until recently, I took this drug called Keppra. It made me
angry, and it caused me to do some terrible things that I
regret. A few years back when I was on the highest dose
the anger was really bad. I punched my mom in the side of
the head, in the temple, while she was driving. She drove
our van into a snow bank because she blacked out. I put

both of our lives in danger. I know myself and I know I wouldn't punch my mom. She tells me all the time she knows it was the drug and that it changes how my brain works. It still doesn't feel good. There is an actual name for this side effect, "Keppra Rage," and my mom kept asking about these side effects. I'm not sure that anyone took her seriously when she tried to explain the level of anger and mental health issues I was experiencing. Keppra has not been good for me and I could not get off the drug without medical assistance because I would have a seizure. Once I had medical support to get off Keppra things changed. Even as we cut that drug back I could feel the anger retreating. When I was finally off it I felt so much better.

When I try to describe the level of anger and rage I feel on this drug, I can't find the words. There's no description for what Keppra does to you. The thing is, even before Keppra, I was always a little fiery, always had a little bit of a temper, but Keppra amps that anger tenfold. It's such a force. You can't stop being angry. You're always angry. You're angry when you wake up, you're angry when you go to bed, you're angry just breathing. You're angry while you're sleeping. I remember when I was on 3,000 milligrams of Keppra and I was angry in my fucking dreams.

Lamotrigine gave me incredible joint pain that eventually went away. The pain made me feel like I was constantly growing, like I was going to be 6 foot 8 or something. My mom packed me in heating pads and gave me Advil to give me relief as I adjusted.

And the fatigue is overwhelming. My mom wakes me to medicate me and the drugs make me sleepy, but then I have to get up and participate in life and I just can't. The anger and fatigue and memory and other stuff, that's enough for another book, almost. When you're a teenager, you're moody and you're tired anyways. You add epilepsy to that ... you have seizures and you wake up tired and then you have the fatigue from the seizure, and then you add depression on top, which makes you tired, and then you add anxiety which makes you... it's just hard to function. I don't know if my fatigue is the drugs, I don't know if it's the depression, I don't know if it's being a teenager or if it's just a mishmash of it all.

It constantly feels like there's someone, and I mean someone heavy, sitting on your back. Pretend that you're on an ice road and you're naked, lying face down and you have to get all the way to one end of the road on your belly. All you have to move yourself from one place to the other is little toothpicks. You drag yourself. That's the only way. That's what it feels like. Things feel insurmountable. Impossible.

**Fear without Shame**

I don't really fear much. I'm not afraid of dying anymore. The thing is, it scares me that I'm not afraid of it. I have told my mom that if I die during a seizure, she needs to know it doesn't hurt. It looks scary I am sure, but it doesn't hurt.

My fear is embarrassment, like having a seizure in public. I know people can urinate or defecate when they have a seizure. Luckily, that's never happened to me, but I have thrown up. I don't want to walk out of high school with puke all over me. I've always had the fear of that, so that's another reason why I hate going to school.

My fears include being embarrassed and people not wanting to be friends with me because of my epilepsy. It's too much to handle. My one friend was saying how she doesn't invite me to hang out with all our friends. We talk all the time and she loves me, but we were talking and I asked, "Why don't you ever invite me to go places with you and our other friends? You always have Snapchat stories of you hanging out with your friends." She said, "Oh, well, we're scared if you have a seizure something might happen and we can't do anything." It is hard not to feel dismissed.

I responded, "It's okay. I'm controlled for the most part." "Well, we'll invite you next time for sure," and they didn't. They were scared. It's a piss off, because I want to be a normal kid. All I want to do is be a normal kid and not have to worry about all this other crap, but here I am worrying about all this bullshit.

I have some fears related to the seizures in public and stuff like that, which are totally legitimate, but I have to deal with the fear other people have about me. It is hurtful and frustrating. So often I sit at home. Fear surrounds me and most of it isn't mine.

J ennifer:
      As a parent, it's very difficult to watch somebody slip

into the abyss, but I've also realized that, while I can support Chiara in this battle, it is her personal battle. She needs to be prepared to show up to that battle in the best possible condition she can be in, and that means she needs to pay attention to her sleep, to what she fuels her body with, to how hydrated she is and to medicine compliance. All of these things, ultimately, are up to her, and it's exhausting as a parent to take on the responsibility of trying to make your child sleep or trying to make your child eat healthy or trying to make your child remember when they're supposed to take their medicines. And sometimes depressed people just don't care. They are drowning in the day-to-day stuff and anything you add on top is too much.

This has been my hardest lesson. This has been the most helpless feeling in the world, because I would trade places with her in a moment to give her the 40 years I've had to live her life fully and completely. I hope that she grows into the understanding that while I can support her with everything I've got, ultimately, she has to decide how she's going to show up on the battlefield. It's very difficult when you're fighting anxiety, depression and epilepsy medication side effects WHILE you are trying to grow and develop. Most fully mature adults would struggle too.

If I can say anything in her defence, it's simply that some days she just can't. Some days, she just can't get out of bed. Some days, she just can't do what you ask of her. She's told me time and time again, "Mom, it's not like I don't want to go to school. I want to go to school. I want to be around my friends. I just can't." I'm not fighting her battle, so I can't possibly know what she's experiencing firsthand. I just know what I see, and I know that sometimes Chiara doesn't let me see the ugly, ruthless side that she's living inside her mind.

I've heard epilepsy being referred to as the disease of anticipation. It's not a matter of if you're going to have your next seizure, it's when, and you live with that anticipation looming over your shoulder. Will it be when you're barrel racing your horse at a competition? Will it be when you're on stage in a youth theatre production? Will it be when you're in the middle of an exam? Will it be when you're sitting in class? Will it be when you're walking through the hallway? Will it be when you're home alone? I just beg everybody to consider, for a moment, what life must be like for people who suffer from epilepsy and the side effects of their medications and the associated mental health issues that come with a diagnosis like this. It is life changing, and it can be a very difficult beast to manage.

Chiara and I have never hidden the fact that she has epilepsy. We speak openly about it to everybody that we meet, and we do this for a few reasons. Mine is particularly selfish. I want the world to know that my daughter has this condition, because if she finds herself in a situation where she needs help but she can't verbalize what she needs, I want the people around her to know that she has this condition so that they can step up and provide her with some sort of first aid and access to medical care.

I also know that the post-ictal phase can be extremely confusing for Chiara, and I have visions of her coming out of a grand mal seizure not knowing who she is or where she is and wandering off panicked into a world that has no idea that she suffers from epilepsy. I imagine what law enforcement would think if they came across her on a bus. If she was confused and disoriented, would they make assumptions? Would they treat her differently because of that? I want to teach the world to be compassionate to people who suffer from these types of invisible conditions, so Chiara and I are not going to hold our tongues. We are going to share everything we can so that we can educate the people around us and keep everybody, including Chiara, safer.

When Chiara's friends come over, if I'm leaving and they're going to be together without me there, I make sure that they know what to do in case of an emergency, not only to help Chiara but also to prepare them so that they are not frightened. I tell everybody to please just call 911, and I'm blessed to have insurance coverage to cover the ambulance costs, because epileptics can get into trouble really fast. There isn't a lot of time to mess around. I don't think there should be shame associated with being an epileptic, but we know there are still stigmas. I don't think that these people should feel like they need to hide a condition that can put their life in danger.

# Chiara:
## The Hospital

**Does it make a difference to you how hospital staff and emergency staff respond to you? How can they make a positive difference when you are hospitalized?**

It makes a massive difference, in my opinion. The staff needs to be professional, and it can hurt when you hear their opinions. For example, I overheard two nurses talking about me when I was in their ward. One was like, "Yeah, no I like her. She's cute." The other was like, "I don't mind her." That set off my anxiety and so I was freaking out over something so little. I know it's little, and I know it's stupid, but it still made me really nervous. I try to be polite and not ask for anything at all, but sometimes I do need help and I am afraid to ask. It really makes a difference if the nurses and hospital staff are friendly.

When I was in emergency last time, I had the best para-medics. They talked to me and they were funny, which is a great distraction. It is scary when your health care profes-sionals are complaining and roughly jamming the IV in your arm and so forth. You really just want to feel cared for and safe. If the health workers are having a bad day, they should try not to take it out on you because you are having a bad day too! I've had that before. Friendly hospital staff is definitely needed. I have called my mom at home to come back to the hospital to help me because I have been too afraid of the medical staff. I also recognize that not all patients are nice to the staff and that is not cool either. I do try very hard to be polite and respectful too.

Another thing that is important to share is that it is often very hard to share what is actually going on. Many times my mom and I have sat in a doctor's office and we try to share what is happening and we may not feel like the doctor is listening. Don't be that doctor. We have come for help but often our slow responses are not because we have nothing to say or share or ask. We have too much to share or say or ask. We are afraid. We are worried. We are so very close to breaking down that to begin speaking is hard. Be patient with us and be kind. You will see only a glimpse of the struggle and you will only see it if you make us feel safe enough to share with you.

**What about a sense of humor from the hospital staff?**

Sense of humor makes everything better. Joshua, if you are reading this, your sense of humour was greatly appreciated. Thanks for calling me out on my sass and taking part in a little smack talk when I was sort of making sense in the ER both times you transported me.

**When you're in the hospital, does it make a difference when your friends come to visit you?**

Yeah, because then you feel like you are loved and it feels less like the world is moving on without you. If people don't come and visit you, you feel like you don't have any friends. Forgotten. Insignificant. Luckily, I did get visitors, so it made me feel better. I know I've had friends who've been in the hospital, and they didn't get any visitors. Even though they have lots of friends, no one came to visit them and that's hard. I have great friends. If you are reading this, thank you for all you do to help me feel loved!

Feeling alone is not fun. Hospital rooms get dark and depressing fast.

# BARREL RACING

## A Poem

We breathe heavy
as they call our names.

The thumping of our hearts become one.
She knows the game, she knows the rules.
So do I.

The other half of me, the one I sit upon,
knows what is coming.
She can hardly contain herself.
I try to calm my nerves,
but I can't.

I feel my chest constrict
and the vomit crawls up my throat.
The newly worked ground smells
deliciously natural and earthy.
It calms me slightly.

Three barrels.
Count them Chiara.

As her back feet dig
into the ground behind us
we soar
picking up the right lead.

The thudding of her hooves on the ground is home.
As we approach the barrel
I ready her for the turn.
Time slows to what feels like forever.
I hear nothing. Nothing.

She rates herself
in my mind I call her a good girl.
I let go of the reins with my left hand
and place it on the horn
firmly.

I squeeze my legs
and turn her tight
around the barrel
with my right hand.
It's perfection.

Time is suddenly spinning
around my head yelling,
"I'm going faster, you better hurry up."

Her gallop is like a rocking ship
swaying me back and forth,
back and forth.
The second barrel
suddenly right in front of me.

I forget everything,
but she doesn't.
She switches leads
slows herself steady.
Her turn is sharp.

My boot grazes the barrel.
We turn and run away quickly.
The barrel starts to sway
PLEASE DON'T FALL! PLEASE DON'T FALL!!
I think to myself.

YES!
The swaying slows,
the barrel is still upright.
I look ahead
Focused

Sailing towards the third,
we are ready;
our favourite barrel.
Almost always perfect in our eyes.

Rate. Horn.
Squeeze. Turn.

Her body feels horizontal to the ground as we move.
She loves it.
We both do.


Time has slowed once again,
we are one.
This feeling,
heaven.
It's a drug that you can't stop chasing.


Sadly, it ends too quickly
but the drug's effects aren't over yet.
It's time to run home.
Where we
belong.


She is in
Full-tilt speed
before I even
know it.
I don't have to ask


The storm that we are,
her hooves -- the thunder of
our bodies -- the spiralling clouds
and me,
the fire that ignites it all


The rapture -- ends
The time -- doesn't matter.
What we feel matters.

And that feeling is
perfection

## THE BREAKING POINT

"She is strong, but she is exhausted" – r.h.sin

*I* was done. I have been at the point lots of times, where I have told my mom I was so tired that I just didn't want to be here anymore. But this time she knew I was really done.

As I shared earlier, my mom arranged for me to meet a young woman who has epilepsy and was now expecting her first child. We sat in Smitty's and I cried as I explained how hopeless I felt. She shared with me that she felt the same way when she was my age, too, but that her life is so beautiful now and she is so thankful she stuck it out. She told me she never imagined she could have everything she dreamed of having. She made me feel like I was not alone in this, that maybe there could be a different future for me than the one I currently saw in front of me. A couple days later, she had her baby and to this day I'm sure that baby waited until she had met with me and gave me some hope and encouragement to hang on to.

But then things got worse again. And whoosh, hope was gone again.

In late October of this year, right after my mom picked me up from drama practice, I had a grand mal in the car. I vaguely remember being on the driveway trying to tell her everything hurt but it wasn't coming out right. I guess that is where my recall disappears so she will have to explain what happened. I ended up enjoying a five day hospital stay. I know things were more serious than usual. I aspirated. I had multiple seizures. I had a reaction to the medication they gave me to stop the seizures.

I remember kind of knowing I had another big seizure after I arrived at the hospital, and I remember trying to tell my mom my arm was so sore where the IV was pumping medicine in me but it was just moans that came out. I was stuck somewhere between two worlds. I guess I was in the trauma room by then, and had already been at the hospital for hours, but I had not recovered from the first seizure when I had the second. It's all messy to me so I will let her explain.

# BORN TO DIE

## A Poem

We were born to live.
We were born to feel the sun on our skin.
We were born to stare at the night sky and wonder.
We were born to love.
We were born to laugh.
The only reason we are here is to LIVE, is it not?
We were born to smile and feel joy.
Weren't we meant to be peaceful?
I thought we were meant to be brave and bold,
but to stay humble.
We were born to live a life filled with lessons
that better us.
We were born to find love,
wherever it may be.
We were born to discover,
seek out new things.
We were born to care.
We were born to be kind and understanding.

We were born to be beautiful on the inside.
Then again, we were also
born to die.

# CRISIS COMES KNOCKING... AGAIN

*J*ennifer:

I picked Chiara up from Drama practice and, this being the height of the Pokémon GO craze, she asked me to chase a Pokémon with her. We stopped at a park, and when I looked at her I noticed she was twitching. I grabbed the Ativan from my purse and tried to get ahead of the seizure but it didn't work. Once I knew she wouldn't be stopping I drove as fast as I could with her belted into her seat so I could get home to have help.

I was literally 500 meters from my front door. Her convulsions got violent and her head tipped back. At this point she aspirated, but I could not un-tip her head, so when I flew into the driveway I laid on the horn to get help, ran around and pulled her half out of the car to tip the fluids away from her throat. I was too late. She was half on the concrete, half in the car, half hooked in the door. My boyfriend ran out and helped me pull her from the car and onto the driveway, and we waited for her to come around.

But she didn't. She moaned and mumbled and slurred and tried to get up and fell. She didn't appear to be coming back. At this point I called 911. Again.

We headed off to the least busy hospital and into the ER we went. She had a great doctor whose daughter actually also has a seizure disorder, so he was very trusting and interested in what I had to say as I stood there with her seizure journal, her bag of meds and my detailed account of what happened. Over the next several hours, Chiara didn't really wake up. She seemed odd. I couldn't really explain it but I told the doctor that something was wrong. He trusted me instead of pushing us back out. He said he knew I knew this disease like no one else, and if I said something was wrong, he would keep investigating. I appreciated his trust in me as a parent.

Moments later, she had another grand mal. I rolled her into the recovery position and yelled for help. Her little room filled with doctors and nurses. Meds were administered and I stood back and watched this all in slow motion. Time blends into the walls.

I can't recall all the details, but they moved her to a trauma room at that time. I called her father because now, I was very unsure of how things were going to play out. This was some brand new, absolutely terrifying territory.

She didn't come back. She remained in a haze between two worlds. She didn't respond to her dad or me. For hours, I watched her and the machines and tried to figure out what all her stats meant. They gave her more meds and she became restless, moaning, and I wondered if she was still in pain. I pulled up her sleeve and saw red streaks running from the IV up her arm. She was having a reaction to the anti-seizure medicine, so they stopped the IV. They wanted to transport her to the main hospital, but needed an ambulance that could handle the IV as she was moved. Now they didn't need that ambulance, and a regular one arrived shortly and off she went to the ER at the other hospital. Neurology assessed her and we waited a patient 27 hours for a bed.

And here is where I think the universe shifted things for her. At 17, she was being prepped to move from pediatrics to adult neuro. On this visit, the neuro team consulted the epileptologist on staff because she was wasn't exactly an easy case to handle. And this is where things began to shift.

New eyes, new hope, right?

Once up on the ward and once she had come out of the seizure stupor she was in, she remained on some new meds but the new doctor also wanted her off Keppra and on a new drug called Brivlera. The only problem was, I had never been able to pull Keppra completely before without her having a seizure. While I was excited about trying something new, I was equally terrified.

After five days, Chiara was released to go home. We had a new Rx and a plan. I left work and we began changing her meds. She slept lots and she was miserable. Her mental health was in the tank. Her memory was like vapour. We had many of the same conversations over and over again.

But, she successfully got off the one drug we both hated; the one drug that changed her personality more than anything else did five years ago. We introduced the new medication, and she didn't have any side effects. She had a few seizure events on the lower dose and then they stopped.

As I write this, she is five months seizure free. The darkness has lifted. The new doctor wondered out loud if the Keppra alone was not responsible for her depression and anxiety. UGH. Five years of that shit and struggle could have been avoided … maybe. We will never know. I am just thankful for a new approach and his understanding that her quality of life was as important as her seizure control.

The winds had shifted. Dare we hope? While you may find it hard to see how I feel grateful for what happened to her in this last hospital stay, I am. It changed her life. It put her on a different path. Believe it or not, in all this I see some blessings.

"No mud, no lotus." - Thich Nhat Hanh


C hiara:
        I eventually left the hospital and tried to get back in the game. Easier said than done. Behind in school. Overwhelmed. Checking back out.

After an argument one morning with my mom about

getting up and making a plan for the day, I sent my mom this message …

"I'm sorry...you're an amazing mom and you're so patient and I need that from you for just a little longer...remember, you're watching the seizures I'm having them...not to say your life is easier because it isn't...our lives are just different kinds of hard."

I think that it is important to think about how my epilepsy impacts others. It is hard on me and it is hard on my mom, but in different ways. It is hard on my grandparents, siblings and cousins, but in different ways. Everyone who loves me carries a little bit of my burden, but they don't live it.

Sometimes you just need to trust your madness and do what you know you need to do, knowing no one can truly understand even if they try their hardest. That's okay... they try and I love them all for it.

## DARKNESS RISING

*I* began to feel a little lighter and definitely less frustrated. I had a hard time finding the words to describe how I felt, but I knew something was changing. However, I am still cautious. I've been on this stupid rollercoaster for years, and I know that what goes up, must come down.

Dare I begin to hope? I know my mom was counting the seizure-free days. I had been having them weekly before I went into the hospital, and she marked them all down in that stupid book where she also records how my sleep was and if I was bitchy. I know she was counting the days, holding her breath and not saying anything to me. I bet she still is counting and she probably always will.

The new doctor said the goal was to get me seizure free and to get me out of bed and into life. I was too afraid to even imagine what that might look like. But things were shifting. Can my story end here, on an upswing?

# RE-ENTRY TO LIVING

"One the storm is over, you won't remember how you made it through, how you managed to survive. You won't even be sure, in fact, whether the storm is really over. But one thing is certain. When you come out of the storm you won't be the same person who walked in. That is what this storm is all about." - Haruki Murakami

*W*ith my seizures now apparently controlled with this new medication, and plans in place to reduce my other medications this summer to lessen the side effects and sedation I still feel, I guess I have to learn what it might mean to be able to live without this heavy weight on my back. Can I put it down?

I had stopped attending school after the last hospital stay, but continued to try to do some work from home as I was able. January term break was quickly approaching and I knew my mom wanted me back in school. I was sort of excited at the thought of finishing things up but also very uncertain.

As I started feeling better, my mom started giving me more space and helped me do some things I have never done before. She dropped me off at a house party and went home and then picked me up when I called later to say it was done. I had space. Experience. I attended the Grade 12 formal. I was taking part in life.

## BULLET PROOF

### A Poem

I am stronger
I have fallen
so many times.
Time and Time again,
scraped my knees,
bashed my face,
bit my tongue,
choked,
burned my face,
and cried and screamed
at the world asking,
"Why?"
"Please just give me a small break!"
"Help me."
I have fallen,
dropped so deep
that I have wanted to give up.
I have wanted to die.
I've begged for it.

But
instead I have risen
from each defeat

Each time I am on the ground,
I get angry
And I choose to grab my enemy
by the ankles and pull
him down so
I can rise triumphant

I've shed more tears of sadness
than of joy
I've felt more pain
than needed.
Epilepsy is like a loaded gun
waiting to be fired
Good thing
I'm bullet proof.

# REBIRTH: IMAGINING THE FUTURE

**"And the day came when the risk to remain tight in the bud became greater than the risk it took to blossum." - Anais Nin**

*D*oes this mean I get to be normal? Do I get to worry about Instagram likes and bad hair days instead? What does a superficial teenage passage look like when you have been fighting demons in the dark for five years?

I struggle to imagine what might be out there for me. I have habits that I need to change. I need to push through some uncomfortable things. I have to do things I do *not* want to do in order to do things I *do* want to do.

Recently, I have started thinking that I have not been thinking big enough about what I can do in the future. Some things have shifted, and I am feeling lost and uncertain about how this all will unfold. If I have learned anything, I have learned nothing is EVER certain.

I have imagined nothingness for so long, it is scary and strange to imagine something. It is weird to think of possibilities. Maybe I am just afraid opportunity will toy with me forever?

I want to travel. I want to see the world. I want a job and I want to contribute and be responsible. I want to step back into real life and off social media and have experiences. I want to sleep less and do more. I want to laugh. I want healthy relationships and simplicity. I want spontaneity, but I also want predictability. Remember, there is freedom in predictability and spontaneity is only fun if you are the one making the choices.

J ennifer:

Hope is a funny thing. It can be incredibly torturous, because on the other side of hope is a deep valley of despair. When thing don't go as you hope and pray, the crash landing can be hard. And if you crash time and time again, you begin to stop hoping. You don't bother with trying. You go through the motions, but you stop attaching any emotional currency to the outcome, because you've take the ride to shitsville too many times. You've had your heart smashed and you've had to witness it in others. You just begin to give up.

You stop believing in hope, but you just can't quite close the door. Because hope oozes in any crack it can .... it gets in, even when you want it to just leave you alone. Hope is a beautiful thing when it delivers. But we are terrified, because we know how hard the fall can be.

So for now, I hold my breath and speak not of what I

dream Chiara can have in her life, but instead pretend I
have no dreams at all. We act like if we do not verbalize
our hopes, they cannot be taken away. But secretly, I sit
and wonder … and pray for all sorts of blessing to fall into
her life in the most remarkable way.

## PAYING IT FORWARD

"One day she decided to gather up all the sad stories she told about her life and release them in a big bonfire. She sent the sparks and ash to the heavens where they were transformed with divine love. She declared the past complete and spread a blanket of love & amnesty over every morsel of her life. "A cheer went up in the heavens and the angels rejoiced. The girl had found her way to her light. And with a giggle and a twirl, she set sail for new adventures." - Laurel Bleadon-Maffei

Here I am, about five months post hospitalization and I have been seizure-free since the second week I was home. That does not mean that everything just got better overnight. I still struggle. I have a lot of catching up to do.

I am still trying to reduce my medications, but the agreement was that we would hold steady and allow me to focus on school and graduation. I really want to be done school so I can figure out how my life is going to look in the next little while.

My mom has told me I need the summer to just be a kid… To go up north and swim in the cold, fresh clear northern lakes. To ride a bike. To learn to drive. To go out with friends. To do things I haven't been able to do. To go back to being 12 and do what I missed along the way.

In the fall, I will look for part-time work as we learn what I can manage and when work will fit in best between medication fatigue.

I am beginning to imagine something greater for myself than I have imagined in a long time. But for now, I am holding my breath, tossing ideas around in my mind but not openly sharing. I am afraid. Uncertain. Holding my breath.

As this journey comes to a close for now, I want anyone reading this book to know that we each have our own struggles to face. If you have not struggled yet, you likely will. I think I initially had this idea that life was fair and I have come to see that is not so, but we can still navigate around things that get in our way of living a good life. On the darkest days, have hope. Just hold on. Just hold on.

# BLOOM

## You are being fertilized.

Just Hold On
Love can come in many forms.
But the love I speak of is like a lotus
as it blooms from the mud.

Disgusting and worthless mud.
But the lotus will bloom from the mud
and bring beauty to it.
But to care for the lotus,
you must also care for the mud.
To care for beauty,
you must also care for ugly.
To care for love,
you must also care for hate.
To love someone,
you must care for all of them.
Everyone has the ability
to bloom like a lotus.

But with the lotus,
there is always mud.
Mud helps the lotus grow.
The mud brings beauty.
Without the mud,
there would be no lotus.
You might be mud right now
But you can bloom my friend.
Just hold on.


If you are deep in the mud right now, these times are not worthless. They are fertilizer for your greatness and for your growth. Know that when you are in the mud, it seems hopeless because you cannot possibly see how beautiful you will bloom, and nor can I. The good will return. You will bloom out of the mud, Just Like the Lotus. I am patiently waiting to see how this all turns out.


"The lotus flower blooms most beautifully from the deepest and thickest mud."
- Buddhist Proverb

# ABOUT THE AUTHOR

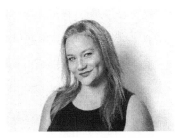

Chiara is 18 years old. She loves horses and spending time outdoors. She graduated from high school in June of 2017 despite missing hundreds of school days due to medication side effects, complications from seizures and severe anxiety and depression.

With almost ten months of stability behind her, she is looking forward to watching her life unfold beautifully.

*If you want to send Chiara a message, feel free to email her through STOKE Publishing.*

stokepublishing@hotmail.com

# AFTERWORD

At time of publication (Oct 2017), Chiara has been stable for almost ten months with the exception of about two weeks where she began experiencing petit mals again. However, her seizures were triggered by something and we had anticipated it. To keep her and others safe, she was not allowed to drive until we saw no evidence of these seizures and her behaviour returned to her new normal.

The return of her seizures, even though anticipated brought back to the surface an increased level of anxiety, fear and questions about her future.

This is an ongoing journey.

Chiara will be entering the work force this fall part time so that we can monitor her energy levels and ensure that she slowly increases her output without incident. With so many variable so manage, change is slow.

As she begins to apply for work we enter a new phase of managing this disorder... Do we tell potential employers when she applies? Or at the interview? Do we risk having her pushed aside out of fear? We can't possible leave them uninformed … we don't feel that is fair to anyone.

How do I prepare her for this next big step into the world?

If you would like to follow Chiara's writing adventures, please join her list here:
https://forms.aweber.com/form/56/63105756.htm

And, should you feel like her words and experience are helpful or provided you with insight, please consider reviewing her work and offering hope, praise, and feedback. I have told her so many times that her experience may help inform others who will then know how to help their loved ones in new ways.


Thank you,

Jennifer (Chiara's Mother)

Made in the USA
Columbia, SC
19 October 2017